I0411433

Getting To The Core Of Apple Cider Vinegar

The Ultimate Guide Book To Apple Cider Vinegar Health Benefits, Home Remedies & More

By: Nicholas Stiles

ISBN-13:978-1482524178

TABLE OF CONTENTS

PUBLISHERS NOTES

Disclaimer

DEDICATION

This book is dedicated to my wife and two boys for their love and support.

PREFACE

Perhaps you are wondering why another book on apple cider vinegar. Apple cider vinegar has been written about for centuries, but the dynamics of the topic continue to change.

One Google search pulls up a litany of clickable links on page after page to learn more about apple cider vinegar. As does a search on Amazon's kindle site – books of every angle on the topic available at the touch of a finger. A check at your local library doesn't produce quite as much information to choose, but any of the books available there lead to the same conclusion as Google or Amazon.

Before you know it, confusion and indecision suddenly show up as the internet user quickly learns the hype surrounding apple cider vinegar makes finding the truth or the facts to be involved, complicated, and confusing. Rather than leaving the search with answers and satisfaction, more "what if's" show up and even fewer answers seem concrete as before they went looking.

The best purpose a new book on apple cider vinegar could serve would be to wade through all the confusion, find what is known, and present it as the most up-to-date, conclusive resource.

This book is to act as a filter through all the information funnelled down to you, to dissect the hype from the truth, to help you learn all that's actually and scientifically known about apple cider vinegar so you, too, can know all there is to know.

Surprisingly, there isn't much to prove or disprove as things stand, but if any evidence exists, we read it, researched it, and found where the conclusions best fit.

Maybe you are hoping to enhance your health by adding a daily intake of apple cider vinegar. Perhaps you currently suffer from a particular ailment that's led you to find out more about apple cider vinegar because you keep hearing it may help you. Or you might have heard about the powerhouse of aide contained within a bottle of apple cider vinegar, and you are curious to learn on a myriad of levels.

Whatever reason brings you here, this book provides your answers and gives you direction. Current, concise, complete answers to address the cloud of mystery surrounding apple cider vinegar are littered throughout the pages of this simple guide.

Well, let's get started. We've dug through the landslide of information, and it's exciting to be ready to share what we've learned with you.

Knowledge makes most things so much easier, doesn't it?

Once a person understands or has the proof to reassure, making decisions and knowing how to proceed becomes simply a matter of weighing what's in the balance rather than an onslaught of confusion.

CHAPTER 1 - BACKGROUND

Apple cider vinegar has gotten quite the reputation as a wonder cure of sorts. People seem to be guzzling it as if it is the fountain of youth, not minding the cringe-worthy flavor or sported floaties.

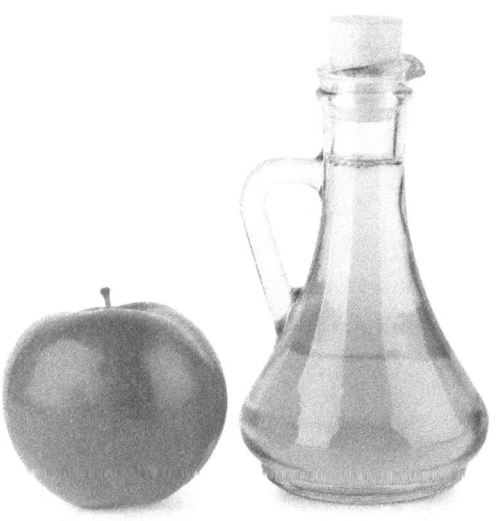

Have an ear infection? Try apple cider vinegar. Diabetes? Gulp some apple cider vinegar. Want to lose weight? Daily apple cider vinegar. A papercut? Apple cider vinegar. Oops, no, probably not that one. Disobedient child? Apple cider vinegar on a spoon! You know . . . that one may have some merit.

Truly there is much to find amazing about apple cider vinegar. For those of you looking to enhance your lives by adding in a swallow or two a day of apple cider vinegar, you'll learn what you can expect based on the gathered data of those who have walked the path ahead.

For those who are suffering a medical ailment and wondering if apple cider vinegar will lessen your symptoms, relieve them altogether, or even provide a cure, the book will highlight what has been proven to support any or all of the above. As much as possible, the book will simply lay out what is known about apple cider vinegar so that you can decide for yourself how you would like to move forward in regards to adding apple cider vinegar into your life.

There is much hype, especially on the internet, surrounding apple cider vinegar. Even just the firm beliefs that people may hold to based on long-term practices contribute to the hype, especially when the foundation of proof has never existed. The frustration in the hype lies in the fact that there is truth immersed in the hype.

Apple cider vinegar is actually very much a reliable remedy to many ailments. To filter helpful information from the propaganda, scientific evidence is required. Or, at least, a large enough number of anecdotal evidence that no one's done a study on to verify medically or scientifically yet.

One thing to keep in mind is that ample proof does exist for several claims made in support of apple cider vinegar's daily use. Scientific evidence being unavailable does not mean studies have proven most or certain claims false. On the contrary, more often than not, the studies have simply just not been done.

Natural substances used for healing are often considered in an alternative health realm, such as in the categories of homeopathy and naturopathy. Not many research resources are excited about funding research on items that fall so closely to hockey "witch doctor" practices or some such other popular stigma for alternative medicines.

Stigma surrounding medicinal approaches not straight out of a pharmacy is still fairly high. When trying to promote research to come to a scientific foundation, it's much simpler for a discovered drug ingredient to be tested than a natural product like apple cider vinegar.

In the meantime, many success stories regarding the use of apple cider vinegar all carry a common thread that is strong enough to show sometimes evidence doesn't have to be necessarily scientifically proven.

When overwhelming evidence exists to support a claim, it would be foolish to dismiss the claim as hype based entirely on lack of scientific support. Things presented as factual in this book which don't have the subsequent backing of medical or scientific proof are being included simply on the basis of vast anecdotal evidence or personal experience.

Hopefully, as time goes by, more factual proof will be discovered to help categorize which claims about apple cider vinegar are true and helpful and which are false and a waste of time and energy.

If you are already accustomed to healthy living and maintaining an on-going self-education is a priority to you, learning what is documented in this book will help you decide if adding apple cider vinegar into your daily regimen is something you want to consider. As knowledge changes with the discoveries over passing time, sometimes the shift in behavior is dramatic, but often changes are gradual with minimal differences.

Chances are, however, that an ailment with little to no resolve among the medical community has led you here. Answers haven't been coming, and you are possibly frustrated with feeling directionless. Apple cider vinegar can help with many medical problems that are left unaddressed or handled via only symptom management. Here is your resource for digging through the hype and finding out what really may hold hope for your future.

CHAPTER 2- DEFINITION

What is apple cider vinegar?

A surprisingly simple process with a surprisingly simple finished product, apple cider vinegar is made directly from apples with a specialized yeast. Organic apple cider vinegar moves the process to a wooden barrel.

Although the word "vinegar" is part of the title of apple cider vinegar, the two substances are really quite different. Vinegar and apple cider vinegar are similar in that both are made via fermenting. Vinegars made from fermented grapes are balsamic. Distilled white vinegar, the standard basic vinegar, is made from a grain base. Rice vinegar, as it's called, is made from rice. Apple cider vinegar is made from apples, following a specific fermenting process.

Apple cider vinegar is fermented twice to become itself. Apple cider is first fermented into hard (alcoholic) apple cider, and then it is fermented a second time to become apple cider vinegar.

Raw, unprocessed, undistilled, organic apple cider vinegar is the only helpful, healthy variation of apple cider vinegar that applies to the suggestions to follow.

Apple cider vinegar is alkalizing to the body, offering also the "mother," whereas distilled vinegar is nutrient-free due to the distillation process. The majority of vinegars are used in cooking, but apple cider vinegar Is the exception as its primary use has become the health related.

There is some history to the process that brought apple cider vinegar to its popularity today, starting with a book by Dr. Jarvis that reached popularity in both the 50's and the 70's. Dr. Jarvis and Dr. Bragg are both medical names closely associated with the popularity of apple cider vinegar, both producing books chock full of remedies and healthy suggestions that all required apple cider vinegar.

Apple cider vinegar is often mixed with honey both for flavor and for added health benefits, but it almost always needs to be diluted with some water to protect the teeth from its acidic potency. When apple cider vinegar is not diluted, a water chaser will ensure the acid leaves the mouth clean.

Crushing the sweetest apples (the higher sugar content is necessary) with some yeast and sugar and allowing the apples to ferment twice will create the "mother." The mother is the debris floating around inside the higher quality apple cider vinegars formed from the pectin and apple residue. It looks something like a webbed, murky mess, but it holds the most nutrients and healing properties. Looking for a mother-heavy apple cider vinegar will assist you in differentiating among the different apple cider vinegars as you determine a high quality carrier. Without the mother, the usefulness of apple cider vinegar decreases to practically nothing.

Making your own apple cider vinegar is a fairly simple process as well, which would allow you to know exactly which organic, sweet apples are involved, keep as much of the mother as possible, and maintain the process in wooden barrels under your own observation. Following is a very reliable recipe, originating with Earth Clinic online (http://www.earthclinic.com):

"Making Cider Vinegar at Home

Two factors require special attention when making vinegar at home: oxygen supply and temperature. Oxygen is spread throughout the mixture by stirring it daily and by letting air reach the fluid through a cheesecloth filter, which is used in place of a regular lid. The temperature of fermenting cider should be kept between 60 and 80 degrees Fahrenheit (F). Lower temperatures do not always produce a usable vinegar, and higher ones interfere with the formation of the "mother of vinegar." Mother of vinegar is a mat that forms on the bottom of fermenting wine that has gone bad. Do not use a metal container when making vinegar; acid in the mixture will corrode metal or aluminum objects. Glass, plastic, wood, enamel, or stainless steel containers should be used for making or storing vinegar. The same holds true for making or storing foods that have more than 1 Tablespoon of vinegar in the recipe.

Steps for Making Cider Vinegar

The following steps must be followed to make a high-quality cider vinegar:

1) Make a clean cider from ripe apples.

2) Change all of the fruit sugar to alcohol. This is called "yeast fermentation."

3) Change all of the alcohol to acetic acid. This is called "acetic acid fermentation."

4) Clarify the acetic acid to prevent further fermentation and decomposition.

Step 1--Making Cider

Cider is made from the winter and fall varieties of apples (summer and green apples do not contain enough sugar). Fruit should be gathered, then washed well to remove debris. Crush the fruit to produce apple pulp and strain off the juice. Use a press or cheesecloth for straining.

Adding yeast to activate fermentation is not essential, but will speed up the process. Special cultivated yeasts are available for this purpose at wine-making shops and biological labs--bread yeasts are not recommended. To make a starter, crumble one cake of yeast into one quart of cider. This makes enough starter for 5 gallons of cider; double the recipe proportionately when making more.

Steps 2 and 3--Making Alcohol and Acetic Acid

Pour all of the liquid into one or more containers to about three-quarters capacity; do not close the lids on the containers. Stir the mixtures daily. Keep the containers away from direct sunlight and maintain the temperature at 60 to 80 degrees F. Full fermentation will take about 3 to 4 weeks. Near the end of this period, you should notice a vinegar-like smell. Taste samples daily until the desired strength is reached.

Step 4--Filtering

When the vinegar is fully fermented, filter the liquid through several layers of fine cheesecloth or filter paper--a coffee filter works well for this. This removes the mother of vinegar, preventing further fermentation or spoilage of the product.

Storing Your Vinegar

The vinegar is now ready for storage in separate, capped containers. Stored vinegar will stay in excellent condition almost indefinitely if it is pasteurized. To pasteurize, heat the vinegar before pouring it into sterilized bottles, or bottle, then place in a hot water bath. In both cases, the temperature of the vinegar must reach at least 140 degrees F to sterilize the product, and should not exceed 160 degrees F. Use a cooking thermometer to ensure the correct temperature is met. Cool the containers and store at room temperature out of direct sunlight."

The varying apple cider vinegars on the market may seem unimportant, but apple cider vinegar is one product where the source matters entirely. Nutrition content differs wildly across the board among apple cider vinegars, and it's important to choose one that is most nutritionally dense. We will discuss this further in Chapter Five.

If you choose to bypass making your own and buy a manufactured product, remember that this is one instance where choosy is better. Look for a dark brown color, a heavy saturation of mother, and the label to declare "organic, raw, unfiltered."

CHAPTER 3- MYTHS

Common beliefs, assumptions, and unsupported practices surround apple cider vinegar. Websites that appear reputable tout lists of nearly every ailment and benefit imaginable.

Potassium, malic acid, acetic acid, and pectin are the nutrient carrier ingredients in most apple cider vinegars. The presence and saturation of each of these differs from manufacturer to manufacturer, sometimes even from bottle to bottle. There is much validity in looking for the darker tinted liquid and the significant presence of the mother.

Some claims being disputed as myths are being disputed purely for lack of scientific evidence, despite ample personal evidence. The testing done on apple cider vinegar is very limited, but dismissing a claim based only on lack of scientific proof may be closing a door on a room full of possibilities.

Now, are there some apple cider vinegar myths that have been disproven on a basis worth noting?

Keep in mind that being disproven is actually vitally different than being "proven" based on lack of proof. Dismissing a remedy suggestion because there isn't enough proof to support it may remove the very thing that would work for you. But if you are more comfortable moving forward with ample evidence provided, it is understandable that you are seeking only remedies with proof. Remember, then, though, that your movement forward will be quite limited.

Some tests try to disprove apple cider vinegar across the entire board based on testing one type and finding conclusive evidence of no nutritional value. One such tester took things a step further, however, and decided consumption of apple cider vinegar not only does literally none of the claimed remedies but also poses a threat to health in general.

Both sides are being pointed out to reiterate the truth that extremes exist in every field, and apple cider vinegar is no different. There are those who believe apple cider vinegar can cure all things – from acne to weight loss. And there are those who swear by a bit each day for nothing very specific.

Just as not enough studies exist to dogmatically prove claims for the usage of apple cider vinegar, neither do any studies exist to rigidly dispute any claims and allow them to become myths. In fact, every title boasting of debunking apple cider vinegar myths only headlines over an article that focused on the inability to prove the vinegar's usefulness. Not one was evidence scientifically or solidly disproving its use.

There are claims that extended use of apple cider vinegar could lower the body's potassium levels. In fact, that claim was found in several places, but no matter how much research dug out, studies or reasoning or proof to back up that hypothesis does not exist. The words "potential for" or "possibility of" always accompanied the threat of lowered potassium. This is pointed out because one of the strongest components to apple cider vinegar that is often credited with having such health impacts is the potassium it contains!

Potassium is to the soft tissues of the body what calcium is to the hard structures of the body. Potassium cleans out arteries, which in turn leads to clearer thinking and an overall general improvement of health. Pure apple cider vinegar, especially made from scratch from sweet apples in wooden barrels, contains a high concentration of potassium.

An evening tonic of honey and apple cider vinegar in a mug of water relieves the body of fatigue and replenishes it with potassium, producing a sensation of vitality.

Along with not knowing enough to taut guaranteed, studied proof of apple cider vinegar's success, there is equally unknown what its risks are or disproven claims. One area to note, however, is the tone of both sides of the myth/evidence battle: On the side of those who claim, even merely anecdotally, to cures undergone via apple cider vinegar there prevails a positive, encouraging hope. On the opposing side of those who highlight the lack of science and study-based proof, the overall tone is sarcastic, belittling, and even mocking.

Sometimes, it is tempting to feel holier than thou, especially in the face of people who seem simpler than a graduated mind. But, all throughout history, such a pattern has existed to show sometimes it is the simpler who may know best. And, sure, sometimes it is the more educated who knows best. Let's just remember a balanced, respectful approach to all people includes those who believe based entirely on something working for them.

The unsupported assumptions happen when people with success stories share what they've experienced with someone else, and that person tries the same approach with the assumption and expectation they will have similar results. Granted, every possibility that they will experience the same success exists, as does – according to evidence – every possibility exist that they will not.

With the status of knowns and unknowns regarding apple cider vinegar, the decision to try it as a medical aide or health enhancement or all out cure remains personal & fairly independent of outside influence.

CHAPTER 4- TRUTHS

Now, on the flip side of the myth-busting journey in the previous chapter, there are many solid truths known about apple cider vinegar. Some results nicely fit scientific tests, some results are premature and show promise, and some show results but don't make sense scientifically.

High cholesterol is one area where science has looked favorably upon apple cider vinegar. A study done on rats (not yet performed on humans) focused on apple cider vinegar consumption in an effort to determine whether or not cholesterol was impacted.

The study's evidence was published in the British Journal of Nutrition in 2006, showing reduced cholesterol levels. The scientists were even able to pinpoint how the apple cider vinegar was affecting the rats in order to produce lowered cholesterol. First, the apple cider vinegar showed action in the liver and then, also in the secretion of the bile acid. Studies such as this show much promise to produce a parallel or, at least, similar conclusion in humans. Since hamsters have a metabolism breakdown similar to humans, researchers are encouraging the next testing to take place with hamsters.

Similarly, rats were studied to see how apple cider vinegar affected high blood pressure. And, again, the findings showed reduced blood pressure levels. The researchers at Bioscience, Biotechnology, and Biochemistry were able to ascertain the acetic acid (typically the most concentrated ingredient in apple cider vinegar) was responsible for lowering the high blood pressure in the rats.

The one medical condition that has been extensively (in comparison) researched is diabetes. Apple cider vinegar and diabetes partner so well, the medical community's attention has been alerted and studies continue to prove the partnership is wise and worth pursuing. Despite being the most encouraging area for progress in regards to scientific proof, the studies and research are yet in their emerging stages. Several studies have proven blood glucose levels are reduced by apple cider vinegar consumption. And one study specifically demonstrated that humans with type 2 diabetes who drank two tablespoons of apple cider vinegar every day impacted their morning levels of blood sugar. The blood glucose levels of the people who took two tablespoons of apple cider vinegar the night prior were lowered four to six percent.

Apple cider vinegar is used for weight loss or weight maintenance by thousands of people. There is some scientific evidence that suggests drinking some apple cider vinegar before a meal encourages feeling full, reducing the amount of food consumed. The studies remain fairly inconclusive without an overwhelming amount of scientific evidence, but research continues in exciting new ways.

Perhaps in the future, the mystery of apple cider vinegar's effects will be more understandable because of findings yet unlearned in its field.

Many non-scientific remedies hold the status among apple cider vinegar users as proven based on widely accepted success. Even just a simple question, "What are your thoughts on apple cider vinegar?" to friends and family will get a multitude of stories of personal success or through-the-grapevine success. Curing a yeast infection with an apple cider vinegar rinse, gargling with apple cider vinegar for a sore throat, placing apple cider vinegar on a cotton ball and bandaging it over a wart, drinking it every morning to maintain diet, drinking it daily for diabetes assistance, curing acne and brightening the skin, and aiding in digestion are all common claims people make and live by.

By far and large, the biggest claim is weight loss. Science continues to "disprove" the claim, but thousands (or more) of people saw apple cider vinegar work in their own bodies to lose the weight and keep it off. Those who take apple cider vinegar several times a day, often just before meals, have found they are able to lose weight and then maintain where they like to stay within their weight goals.

Critics of the apple cider weight loss diet note there is typically not a lifestyle change or diet adjustments outside of the apple cider intake, which constitutes a "fad" diet and brings about no real change. There is truth to that assessment, of course, but if losing weight was the person's only goal and he or she achieved that goal via the use of apple cider vinegar, it only makes sense that 1) they'd believe completely in its effectiveness and 2) continue to drink it daily.

On the outside of the body, apple cider is often used to rinse the hair as a final rinse in the shower to add shine. The acidity of the product helps strip build up from the strands of hair, allowing the hair to regain its body and shine.

Many, many people have personal success stories regarding apple cider vinegar and warts. Even plantar warts, on the sole of the feet, have responded quickly and thoroughly to regular application of apple cider vinegar. One sceptic took it upon himself to personally test several of the theories projected to him regarding apple cider vinegar. Not one proved differently in or on his own body as was proclaimed to him in the first place, but the biggest impact to him was the way his plantar wart responded and disappeared so quickly. He had a history with plantar warts and was accustomed to using the standard over-the-counter, acid-based solutions that kill all the skin it touches, wart included. The apple cider vinegar, whether or not it touched healthy or unhealthy skin, killed only the plantar wart. He was impressed both with the observance of only the wart dying but also the speed by which it happened. Within a week, his wart was entirely dead, and he was able to remove it on his own. Now, often, plantar warts have gone undetected for an extensive period of time, and he did not specify the age or size of his, but the process of death and removal of the viral growth, if apple cider vinegar works for you, could be a variable timetable.

There has also been solid success documented for skin care on a daily regimen. A sort of tonic made from diluted apple cider vinegar can be used as toner to heal acne and fade scars. The same solution works well as an after shave. These are uses just recommended as helpful.

Another method useful for acne is to begin by steaming your face over a pan of boiling water, with a towel draped over your head to keep the steam channelled to your face. The steam will loosen grease, dirt, and other build up. Pat your skin with apple cider vinegar on a cotton ball to remove the loosened debris. Repeat the steaming & apple cider vinegar patting twice. Have a small dish of apple cider vinegar chilling in the fridge for when you complete the face cleaning, so you can pat the chilled apple cider vinegar on your cleaned skin, closing the pores and toning your skin. Do this deep clean approximately once a week.

For those who suffer from a sunburn, relief is found in soaking in a bath that has a good amount of apple cider vinegar dumped in with the water. Another use widely found to bring relief is using apple cider vinegar as you rub your muscles or your feet. Even bug bites in the summer lose some of their sting or itch after apple cider vinegar is applied to them.

Food poisoning, as an extreme digestion issue, and ongoing digestive issues can often be alleviated or greatly lessened by adding a tablespoon or two to a glass of water. Both acid reflux and constipation have responded to ingesting apple cider vinegar. Stomach spasms and diarrhea are sometimes relieved by sipping little bits of apple cider vinegar. As a prevention for indigestion, if you know you are about to consume a food that irritates your stomach, prepare an apple cider vinegar tea mixture of one tablespoon of apple cider vinegar, one tablespoon of honey in a mug of warm water, and drink it half an hour before the meal. Another way digestion is improved is to prepare one tablespoon of water with two drops of apple cider vinegar. Put the mixture into your mouth, holding it for a few seconds. The pause will allow the mouth to create more saliva, an important digestive juice. Starches begin to digest right in the mouth because of the saliva. Once the apple cider vinegar is swallowed, it also aides in the stomach creating more digestive fluids.

As far as drinking apple cider vinegar, though there are enough claims to fill pages and books, there are several that stand out above the rest due to the sheer number of anecdotal evidence available.

Your joints, if they are achy and arthritic, stand a good likelihood of responding to the antioxidant and anti-inflammatory properties of apple cider vinegar. Calcium-based organisms, such as bones and teeth, can benefit from apple cider vinegar's ability to extract calcium from your diet. However, the apple cider vinegar needs to be diluted when orally consumed because its highly acidic nature can actually take its toll on the teeth themselves as it passes them in the mouth.

After a good workout, drinking a mix of water and apple cider vinegar perks your muscles back up and helps ease the weariness and muscle tension. The amino acids in the apple cider vinegar helps defeat the lactic acid built up in the body and released form a workout.

Just as gargling with apple cider vinegar can relieve a sore throat, it can also effectively rinse your teeth and act as a whitening agent. Be very attentive to the condition of your teeth as the acid in the apple cider vinegar can begin to be too harsh, draining calcium from the teeth and lightly wounding the gums.

A very popular use of apple cider vinegar is while undergoing a whole body detox. A large number of detoxification plans center around apple cider vinegar. Its high levels of potassium clarify the body and can help clear sinus infections, yeast infections, sore throats, and there are even claims it helps clear allergies.

Hiccups, for some, stop almost immediately from a direct spoonful of apple cider vinegar.

The same honey/apple cider vinegar hot water tea concoction has helped an untold number of people achieve rest and calm as they prepare to enjoy how it also assists in a solid night of sleep.

If leg cramps haunt you, making the hot water, apple cider vinegar, honey tea with an extra tablespoon of apple cider vinegar has shown to ease the debilitating night time leg cramping.

Acid reflux even benefits from apple cider vinegar, which is one of the areas not quite logical at first. To cure acid you would use acid? But the concept of the weak stomach causing acid reflux in the first place is what this claim stems from. Drinking apple cider vinegar for acid reflux actually builds the strength of the stomach, enabling the stomach to properly function. Hence, acid reflux is eliminated.

Sometimes a cleanse is centered on a body part, and apple cider vinegar aides in the cleanse.

For the gall bladder, apple cider vinegar encourages gall stones to exit through the bowel movements by creating and ingesting a special mixture of juice, oil, the vinegar. Using an 8-oz glass, mix one part pure olive oil (only olive oil) with two parts pure apple juice and add one tablespoon of apple cider vinegar. On the first day, drink this mixture three separate times, but be sure you don't eat any food. For the second day, you take the mixture twice, and you may drink all the apple juice you'd like, but no water or any other liquid or food. For breakfast on the third day, make a large salad of raw cabbage, carrots, celery, beet root, tomatoes, and lettuce. For a dressing, mix apple cider vinegar and olive oil well and pour over the salad. Steamed greens are encouraged for the third day as well.

Many people have found that eating dairy products causes mucus conditions on an ongoing basis in their lives. If the idea of living without dairy is too much, relief from the post-nasal drip and sinus infections can sometimes be found by drinking a glass of water that has a teaspoon of honey and two teaspoons of apple cider in it every morning, before eating. During the day, one more glass like this is a good idea too.

Kidney stones often dissolve when you fight them with large salads of cabbage, carrots, celery, beet root, tomatoes, green onion, parsley, and cucumbers smothered in apple cider vinegar. Follow the salads up with prunes, raisins, and apples.

On the opposite end of the weight spectrum, an underweight individual is often deficient in enzymes needed to digest and use the foods they eat. No matter how much fat or protein is consumed, the body processes it the same way because it is unable to absorb what it needs to gain weight. To achieve a healthy weight and activate or provide the necessary enzymes, drink a glass of water in the morning that has two teaspoons of apple cider vinegar, one drop of iodine, and one teaspoon of honey in it.

All of these uses, and so many more, have ample anecdotal evidence to support each one being worth a try. However, if your condition is such that a medical doctor is involved, it would probably be wise to consider what he or she is suggesting first or consult with him or her about adding apple cider vinegar into your existing health regimen. If you are free, both medically from your doctor's observation and personally from worry, then seeing if apple cider vinegar can bring relief or a total answer or improvements in any way is worth considering based on the vast anecdotal support.

Bear in mind, however, that every person is unique. You may see no change or have no response, you may only see a little change, you may experience the same results you read or hear about, or you may even have results that are greater than what you heard or expected. The only way to find out is to try!

Follow tested and tried guidelines and amounts, make sure you rinse your mouth with water after ingesting or rinsing with apple cider vinegar, and observe the changes closely as you embark on trying apple cider vinegar for whatever various ailments or improvements.

Those who are already healthy and only looking to enhance their current health may notice the fewest effects. Those who are looking to eliminate specified issues, such as warts or acid reflux, will have an easier time pinpointing success because their focus is in one area. Those who are trying to lose weight have a measureable way to see if apple cider vinegar is working for them. And those who have debilitating illness may or may not see great change since they have the greatest need.

Whatever the case, apple cider vinegar remains largely unstudied but with ample personal proof, some scientific proof as well, to give evidence it is worth considering and trying for the many ailments claimed to find relief under its influence.

CHAPTER 5- ACCESSING APPLE CIDER VINEGAR

Earlier, we discussed the many different varieties available on the market for apple cider vinegar. Every grocery store carries at least one variety, and normally the more popular, convenient apple cider vinegars are not the ones that carry nutritional value. In fact, buying an apple cider vinegar from next to a distilled vinegar, both wearing off brand labels is really just a waste of time. You might as well buy the distilled stuff next to it.

Like most other things, you pay for you get when it comes to apple cider vinegar.

Many varieties of apple cider vinegar in pill form also exist, but research of ample amounts exists that not only are the pills nowhere near as effective as the liquid, but the adverse effects of the pills are worth noting, especially the common esophageal burn just from swallowing the pills.

To find a high quality apple cider vinegar, a grocery store is not typically a great start for looking. Vitamin or supplement stores, health food stores, and other such speciality grocers carry a wider offering. Usually the types these places carry are also all of a high enough caliber to assist you in your goal.

If the label claims it is raw, organic, unprocessed, undistilled, then you've got a great starting place. Just compare, visually, the variations that share the former qualifications. Look at the mother, the deepness of the brown color, and compare the size bottle to the size of the mother. Try to gauge the best product for your dollar.

Pricing for apple cider vinegar changes rapidly, beginning at just a couple dollars and escalating quickly up to twenty or thirty dollars.

For dosing instructions, as discussed in the chapter prior, diluted solutions of apple cider vinegar and water work well for external uses. The muscle rub, acne toner, hair rinse, and other similar uses could be mixed ahead of time in containers that fit in your medicine cabinet or on your bathroom shelf. The hot tea concoction is a fairly standard one tablespoon each of honey and apple cider vinegar, but a few situations call for a more intense dosing of the apple cider vinegar into that mix. Remember, when taking apple cider vinegar orally or using it in your mouth and spitting it back out, always rinse with water afterwards to protect your teeth's enamel from the acid.

Not only does mixing the apple cider vinegar with water or juice or even wine, or adding honey to it and then drinking it as tea in warm water, help the flavor, it aides in a buffer for your body when a straight application of apple cider vinegar would be harsh, either internally or externally.

For specific dosing instructions, most of the anecdotes concerning apple cider vinegar include the measurements or suggested ratios.

Below are some home remedies, some of them already mentioned in the previous chapter, put into an organized list for easier comprehension and access:

Sore throat:

Gargle with ACV; rinse with water.

Dull hair:

Rinse with a mix of ½ ACV and ½ water.

Wart // Plantar wart:

Apply a cotton ball wet with ACV directly to affected skin; secure w duct tape; leave overnight. Repeat until wart is dead and removable or falls off.

Weight loss:

2-3 times a day, typically before meals, drink a shot of ACV quickly chased by water.

Acne:

Tonic of 50/50 ACV & water applied directly to skin.

Drink 1 – 2 tablespoons a day in water.

Muscle aches:

Tonic of 50/50 ACV & water applied directly to skin.

Yeast Infections:

Solution of 50/50 ACV and water used as a gentle wash and douche.

Acid Reflux:

Warm water containing 1 tbsp ACV, 1 tbsp honey.

High cholesterol:

Drink 1 – 2 tablespoons of ACV daily; rinse with water.

High blood pressure:

Drink 1 – 2 tablespoons of ACV daily; rinse with water.

Diabetes:

Drink 2 tablespoons of ACV before bed.

Hiccups:

Spoonful of ACV directly in mouth, followed by drinking water.

Sunburn:

Add cup of ACV to bath water.

Bug bites:

Rub ACV directly onto bites.

Trouble sleeping:

Hot water w 1 tbsp honey & 1 tbsp ACV before bed.

Leg cramps:

Hot water w 1 tbsp honey & 1 tbsp ACV.

Body Detox:

1- 3 tablespoons ACV diluted in water daily.

Digestive issues – including stomach spasms, indigestion, diarrhea, food poisoning:

1-2 tablespoons ACV in 8 oz of water or 1 tablespoon ACV, 1 tablespoon honey in warm water or 1 tbsp water w 2 drops ACV held in mouth for few seconds.

Aching joints, aching muscles:

1-2 tablespoons ACV in water.

Foot fungus:

¼ cup ACV in warm water, soak foot.

Washing fruits & vegetables:

1 part ACV to 3 parts water, soak fruits & veggies, let dry, store in covered container in fridge – no mold & freshness lasts longer.

Fruit Fly Trap:

In small bowl, pour straight ACV, cover w tinfoil, poke tiny holes in tinfoil. Traps gnats or fruit flies.

Gallbladder Cleanse or Kidney Stones:

Follow specified instructions in Ch 4.

Dairy exposure Mucus Control:

8 oz glass of water, 1 tsp honey, 2 tsp ACV, each morning & each afternoon.

Weight Gain/Enzyme Regulation:

8 oz water, 1 tsp honey, 2 tsp ACV, 1 drop iodine, each morning.

Swimmer's Ear:

Drop warm ACV into ear canal, place half cotton ball in ear to hold liquid.

Sinus Infection:

2 tablespoons ACV in 8 oz water until subsides, then 2 teaspoons instead.

Chapter 6- Advantages and Disadvantages

After reviewing all the research, what seems to be the case is when most people sought apple cider vinegar to cure an ailment, they were pleasantly surprised their overall health increased. The many advantages they found to daily consumption of apple cider vinegar caused them to incorporate the liquid as a permanent fixture in their diets. Even after their specific condition improved or disappeared altogether, the changes throughout the rest of their bodies were significant to the degree that stopping the apple cider vinegar seemed foolish.

However, there are very real disadvantages and side effects for some people as well.

If you are not careful to rinse the apple cider vinegar from your mouth after ingesting it, whether diluted or not, the enamel on your teeth can easily begin to erode from the highly acidic nature of the liquid. Even just the gums can become irritated after repeated contact with apple cider vinegar.

There is a chance apple cider vinegar can interfere with your body's ability to absorb and correctly process medications you are on. There's also the risk of, with repeated exposure, the acid could cause lower bone density and less potassium absorption. This statement is not supportable by any medical or scientific evidence, but it was mentioned enough that we would be remiss not to include it at least at the level of knowing it's been said.

Many people report new levels of energy and a clarity of mind after drinking apple cider vinegar regularly.

The advantages and disadvantages, much like what is known or not known, about apple cider vinegar vary person to person.

One advantage of apple cider vinegar is its accessibility, cost, and ease of administration. One disadvantage is the many varieties available, causing a pause to do a little research to determine which one to purchase.

Another advantage is apple cider vinegar is something you can make yourself, allowing control of the ingredients and process to be yours and under your supervision.

CHAPTER 7- LIMITATIONS

Most people groups are well suited to the limited intake and use of apple cider vinegar.

There are limitations, however, that need to be clearly delineated.

Drugs such as diuretics, insulin, or Digoxin can interact with apple cider vinegar in a detrimental way in the body. Particularly, doctors see the possibility for lowered potassium in the blood when these medications combine with apple cider vinegar in the body. Lowering potassium is usually dangerous, or at least unhealthy.

On the twist side, if apple cider vinegar has a reaction with these drugs in the body, then the claims from the outcry of "Myth! Myth!" lose more footing as well. Affects, whether negative or positive, are still affects, meaning apple cider vinegar is not a placebo or akin to drinking merely water.

Apple cider vinegar is highly acidic. Although the theory behind using the acidic liquid is to strengthen the stomach and combat indigestion and acid reflux, doctors continue to warn that repeated exposure to apple cider vinegar may worsen such conditions.

As discussed in Chapter Six, some negative side effects can occur. One medical site even claims consuming apple cider vinegar can cause difficulty breathing, facial swelling, pain in the throat, and hives. Pain in the throat we've addressed, along with the repeated advise to always chase apple cider vinegar drinks (whether diluted or not) with water. The other claims were as unsubstantiated as several of the success stories.

Heart medication or diabetic medication, as mentioned a few paragraphs earlier, may not mix well with apple cider vinegar. The vinegar could interfere with the medicines, hampering their effects, so check with your doctor before you incorporate apple cider vinegar into your life.

Commercially produced apple cider vinegar should also be avoided as it could contain harmful ingredients or simply be ineffective as a product.

If you have low potassium, osteoporosis, diabetes, or heart disease, make sure you talk with your doctor or consult with your medical team before you use apple cider vinegar in your diet or supplementally. The drugs you take for your existing condition(s) may be compromised or even worsened by the apple cider vinegar.

Vinegars contain chromium, altering insulin levels, and necessitating change in your medication for diabetes. The chromium, in this case, is a helpful way to need less diabetes medication as the insulin levels respond, but your doctor should know so he or she may adjust your medication dosages.

So, similar to the specific claims (namely, four) on apple cider vinegar that are proven and scientifically supported, the areas of limitation are also few but scientifically supported.

Information such as both of these is very helpful when trying to decide about incorporating apple cider vinegar into your health regimen. You now know what is specifically known based on science, what is specifically known based on anecdotal evidence, and what is specifically known to contain risk based on science.

CHAPTER 8- CASE STUDIES, ANECDOTES

So far, throughout the book, a few case studies and anecdotes have been briefly introduced. However, truthful, believable apple cider vinegar patrons have little blurbs that created lifetime fans of the liquid from their experiences.

Stephanie soaks her feet in an apple cider vinegar and water foot soak to rid her feet of fungal infections.

Bekah's parents drink grape juice and apple cider vinegar every morning to help their digestion throughout the day.

Several women rave about the success they swear by when they have a yeast infection and use an apple cider vinegar douche to kill the candida.

Colleen's great-grandma, who died at 103 years old, drank a hot toddy every night before bed. Her hot toddy was simply apple cider vinegar and honey in hot water.

The weight loss stories are far, far too numerous to count. Person after person recounts the personal struggle to lose weight and then encountering apple cider vinegar only to discover great and permanent success.

Kristina takes a teaspoon every morning to speed her metabolism.

Jill uses it to treat urinary tract infections and whenever she feels a virus coming.

A handful of people interviewed use apple cider vinegar to treat swimmer's ear and remember doing so as children as well.

Jim's uncle drinks a couple spoonfuls before he eats, insisting his appetite decreases substantially when he does.

As soon as she feels a cold coming on, Sarah brews a cup of herbal fruit tea, adds three tablespoons of honey and one tablespoon of apple cider vinegar and drinks it as hot as she can stand it. A few cups of that brew and her cold is zapped. She swears by it.

These first-person interview results mirror exactly the thousands identical to them all across the internet or daily interactions with others. Try just asking your friends and family what sort of success they've experienced with apple cider vinegar. Most likely the majority will have something, if not more things, to share with you right away. Apple cider vinegar has been around for centuries and used for just as long to remedy all sorts of conditions. Personal recounts abound in practically any avenue you try. The internet, published books, conversation, etc all offer more stories of success.

CHAPTER 9- CONCLUSION

Made from one of the healthiest whole foods on the planet, apple cider vinegar is comprised of extra sweet apples that have been crushed and paired with specialized yeast. Fermentation into a hard cider results, and then a second fermentation process is done to achieve vinegar – apple cider vinegar, to be exact.

All through the years, apple cider vinegar has enjoyed mass public acclaim for doing great good to conditions the medical community typically has little reliable success in, such as indigestion, reflux, skin viruses, cholesterol & blood pressure, and many more.

Recently, apple cider vinegar has come under scrutiny and attack, with an outcry for medical studies and scientific proof to substantiate the anecdotal claims paving the way of the ample success stories. Very few studies have taken place, with even fewer helpful, conclusive results. Some claims now have scientific proof, but most do not. Some health conditions need monitoring when considering using apple cider vinegar.

For the most part, however, apple cider vinegar remains unscathed by the dissenters and naysayers. The myth-busters continue their work at about the same pace as the scientific-proof followers continue theirs. In the meantime, the majority of people believe in apple cider vinegar on the merit of their own experience and success.

With the known myths exposed, the known truths exposed, and the conclusion of anecdotal evidence remaining the strongest proponent of the use of apple cider vinegar, the decision is in your – the reader's – hands.

Apple cider vinegar has lived its existence accepted as a natural remedy and health enhancer. Normally, debunkable theories are, in fact, debunked long before this length of time has passed. Every study and research investigation opens the door wider to discovering what could become more factual data, for either side of truth or myth, based on science.

The charts and facts and evidence or lack of evidence throughout this book show you clearly how to approach the differing situations where apple cider may or may not enhance your life. Risks, minimal or not, are defined.

As you embark on your journey with apple cider vinegar, keep this resource as a reference to use over and over again. Hopefully, science and research will come together to provide the data for Edition Two, where the current information at that time will be even more clarifying and encouraging.

Best of luck with every decision, attempt, and belief!

ABOUT THE AUTHOR

After researching, reading books, and speaking with several people all on the topic of apple cider vinegar, Nicholas Stiles has decided to write this book because his main goal was to make a resource where all the confusion cleared and answers, as best as they exist, are given. Getting to the Core of Apple Cider Vinegar exists as a catch-all resource to help educate the public without bogging them down with confusion or dismissal.

Within the pages of the book, the problem Nicholas is trying to solve, of the confusion surrounding apple cider vinegar's vast claims to health, is approached in every perspective. He dissects why there is so much hype, what constitutes believability, the truth of scientific testing occurring or not occurring, and support based on evidence rather than lack of support being the inability to produce evidence. He shows where there is actually less of a problem and more of a solution without standard data available for support. Empowering the reader with logic and truth is what allows them to read the book and come to the conclusion of making a choice.

www.ingramcontent.com/pod-product-compliance
Lightning Source LLC
Chambersburg PA
CBHW070510290526
45790CB00003B/1179